CBD HEMP OIL 101

The Essential Beginner's Guide To
CBD and Hemp Oil to Improve
Health, Reduce Pain and Anxiety, and
Cure Illnesses

Tommy Rosenthal

REVIEWS

Reviews and feedback help improve this book and the author.

If you enjoy this book, we would greatly appreciate it if you were able to take a few moments to share your opinion and post a review on Amazon.

Table of Contents

Introduction

What do you think about when you hear the word cannabis?

For many, the image that comes to mind is that of people getting high as they smoke a big joint and listen to Bob Marley songs.

It's a bit like: what do you think about when I say: 'Amsterdam'?

However, as any local can confirm, Amsterdam has so much more to offer than weed and coffee shops.

It's the same with cannabis: it is most known for the plants that contain lot of THC, which is the chemical that gets you high. But if you take the time to look a little bit closer, you'll find a lot of other chemicals in there that actually have very *beneficial* health effects.

The main one is CBD, which is short for cannabidiol. CBD is the main component in CBD Hemp Oil.

CBD is a chemical compound found in the cannabis plant. In this book, you will learn about the powerful healing effects CBD Hemp Oil can have.

But I want you to be on board from the very beginning, and address the biggest concern you may have on this first page.

Let's get one thing straight: **hemp *is not* marijuana**.

The difference?

Marijuana gets you high. Hemp doesn't.

The confusion comes from the fact that both marijuana and hemp come from the same plant species: *cannabis*.

The cannabis plants contain a lot of so-called cannabinoids. What are they? Cannabinoids are chemicals in the cannabis plant. They give the cannabis plant its medical and recreational properties.

The two most important cannabinoids are:

- THC (Tetrahydrocannabinol)
- CBD (Cannabidiol)

THC is the chemical that gets you high. It is the main component in marijuana.

CBD, on the other hand, does not get you high. Research has actually shown that CBD even *reduces* the psychoactive effects of THC. Which is why marijuana farmers have cultivated plants with high amounts of THC, but *low* amounts of CBD

Only recently, CBD has been found to have profound positive effects on the health of people that were at a loss for medical treatment. For example, there are cases of children whose severe epilepsy seizures greatly diminished after taking CBD Hemp Oil, when nothing else had worked for them for years.

The field of science that researches the health effects of CBD is young and very exciting. It comes with its challenges, because of the stigma it has that it's a psychoactive drug. But as you will quickly learn, this couldn't be further from the truth! CBD <u>does *not* get you high</u>, and has <u>no</u> other <u>psychoactive effects</u>.

So, CBD is the main component of industrial hemp.

Industrial hemp is a group of cannabis plants within the cannabis sativa category. These are thin, tall plants.

Hemp is considered one of the oldest domesticated crops we know of. It is a very versatile crop: it has been used for textiles, cordage and paper for millennia. Nowadays, its seeds and flowers are also used in health foods and organic body care. CBD Hemp Oil is just one example of such use.

For a plant to be called industrial hemp, not only should it be a cannabis sativa plant, it also needs to meet the following requirements:

- Very low THC percentage: no more than 0.3% (recreational cannabis can contain 20+% THC)
- Rich in CBD

The traces of THC in these plants are so low that there is no chance of you getting high (or having any other psychoactive experience) when you consume any CBD Hemp Oil.

Now that we're clear on that, what *does* CBD Hemp Oil do?

I'm glad you asked! That's what this book is all about.

In this book, you will learn everything you need to know about:

- the ins and outs of CBD Hemp Oil, and

- its purported health benefits

If you are a newbie to CBD Hemp Oil, you have come to the right place.

At the completion of this book, you will have a good understanding of:

- how CBD differs from THC
- the therapeutic effects using CBD Hemp Oil
- how you can start using CBD Hemp Oil and improve your own sense of well-being.

I hope you are excited! Let's get started, shall we?

Chapter One: What Is CBD?

Key Takeaway: Negative perception regarding cannabidiol continues to decline, particularly as its positive effects are unmasked. What exactly is this compound and why is it becoming the next big thing among those looking for natural treatments?

As you learned in the Introduction, Cannabidiol or CBD is a chemical compound found in the cannabis plant. The plant itself contains about 113 active cannabinoids, and cannabidiol is considered a major phytocannabinoid making up about 40% of the cannabis plant's extract.

In recent years, scientific studies have shown the many medicinal effects of cannabidiol. Moreover, its nonpsychoactive characteristics and lack of interference with psychological and psychomotor functions have also been extolled by researchers.

When the subject is cannabis, most people associate it with the widely popular use of the plant as a recreational drug. Hence, compounds in the plant such as cannabidiol are immediately viewed as potentially inducing a feeling of being "high". However, cannabidiol does not cause this feeling in users at all! Rather, it has been shown to all the following effects:

- anti-inflammatory
- antioxidant
- analgesic
- antidepressant
- anti-tumoral
- anti-psychotic, and
- anxiolytic.

Cannabinoid Cell Receptors

Cannabidiol is found mostly inside the resin glands or trichomes of cannabis. CBD, along with other cannabinoids in the plant, binds itself to the cells' cannabinoid receptors, which are primarily found in the body's central nervous system as well as other organs, including the skin, digestive system, and the reproductive organs. The body's cell receptors collectively form a network called the endocannabinoid system.

Endocannabinoid System (ECS)

The endocannabinoid system or ECS is a neurotransmitter system responsible for many regular body functions and feelings, including:

- memory
- motor control
- mood
- reproduction
- immune function
- appetite
- sleep
- pain reception, and
- bone development.

The ECS also regulates the body's energy balance or homeostatic functions. When ingested, cannabinoid appears to interact with the body's ECS, causing the therapeutic effects reported by users of CBD Hemp Oil and other CBD products.

How CBD differs from THC

Cannabidiol is different from another compound also found in the cannabis plant, tetrahydrocannabinol or THC.

THC is the major psychoactive agent in cannabis, and is mainly responsible for that "high" that cannabis users experience when using cannabis recreationally. THC's side effects include:

- lethargy
- decrease in body coordination
- postural hypotension, and
- slurred speech.

Others may also experience hallucinations, mood swings, behavioral changes, paranoia, dizziness, fatigue, or feelings of inebriation when ingesting THC.

That is not to say that THC has not been researched or utilized for medicinal or scientific purposes as well. THC has been formulated into dronabinol and is available by prescription in the United States and Canada, among other countries. Dronabinol is currently being used to treat anorexia or other eating disorders in HIV/AIDS patients, and to control nausea or vomiting experienced by cancer patients who are undergoing chemotherapy.

THC is also an active ingredient in nabiximols, a botanical drug prescribed for people suffering from multiple sclerosis. This drug was approved in the United Kingdom in 2010 to relieve neuropathic pain, overactive bladder function, spasticity, and other effects of multiple sclerosis.

So, THC and CBD both interact with the body's cellular receptors, but the effects are markedly different. Aside from the lack of psychoactive effects in CBD, it also

- balances out or counteract anxiety.
- has antipsychotic effects, unlike THC which can trigger or exacerbate psychosis or hallucinations.
- has – perhaps the most noteworthy – a positive effect on wakefulness.

The Case For CBD: Charlotte's Web

Cannabidiol and its medicinal use broke into mainstream consciousness in 2013, when the case of a baby named Charlotte Figi made headlines. Charlotte, along with her twin Chase, was born October 18, 2006 to Matt and Paige Figi. The twins were born perfectly healthy, but after a few months it became apparent that Charlotte was suffering from a medical condition of some sort.

One day, Charlotte suddenly started having a seizure. She was laying on her back on the floor, with flickering eyes. That first seizure lasted about half an hour, and Matt and Paige rushed their baby to the hospital.

In a CNN article that covered the story, Paige recalled that they weren't calling it epilepsy. They thought it was just a random seizure. They examined Charlotte in every possible way (MRI, EEG, etc.), but found nothing. Ultimately, they were sent home.

However, over the next few weeks, Charlotte would continue to get seizures, some often lasting two to four hours. Hospital tests could not find anything, and the doctors could not figure out what was going on. "*They said it's probably going to go away,*" Paige said. "*It is unusual in that it's so severe, but it's probably something she'll grow out of.*"

After many more tests and frequent seizures, a doctor diagnosed Charlotte with a rare intractable epilepsy called Dravet Syndrome. This form of epilepsy is different in that the epileptic seizures cannot be controlled by any medication. Charlotte was being treated with seven types of drugs, including barbiturates and benzodiazepines, but the seizures were still occurring.

"*At 2, she really started to decline cognitively*," Paige said. "*Whether it was the medicines or the seizures, it was happening, it was obvious. And she was slipping away.*"

They also took Charlotte to a Dravet specialist in Chicago who recommended a ketogenic diet, high-fat and low-carb, used mostly for epilepsy patients. The diet induces the body to produce more ketones which are the body's natural chemicals against seizures. The diet controlled Charlotte's seizures, but not without adverse side effects such as bone loss, compromised immune system, and even behavioral effects.

When her parents saw her eating pine cones and other stuff outside, they asked themselves: is this treatment, with all its unpleasant side effects, truly beneficial?

Matt was desperate, and he began researching online for other possible solutions. He found an online video showing a boy in California also diagnosed with Dravet Syndrome and being treated using a strain of cannabis that was low in THC and high in CBD. The treatment was working to control his seizures.

Charlotte was already five years old around this time, and Colorado had only recently approved medical marijuana. Matt and Paige decided it was worth a shot, but they needed two doctors to sign off on their daughter's medical marijuana card.

After receiving countless rejections, they finally got in touch with Dr. Margaret Gedde, who agreed to meet with them. Even though Charlotte would have been the youngest in the state to apply for the card.

Dr. Gedde signed off on Charlotte's medical marijuana card. *"Charlotte's been close to death so many times, she's had so much brain damage from seizure activity and likely the pharmaceutical medication,"* Gedde said. *"When you put the potential risks of the cannabis in context like that, it's a very easy decision."*

Another doctor, Alan Shackelford, was hesitant because of Charlotte's age, but eventually signed off because of the desperate situation. He felt that all other treatment options had been exhausted, and cannabis was their only remaining option.

They located a marijuana dispensary in Denver selling a strain called R4, with very low THC and high CBD. A friend extracted the CBD oil from the cannabis, and after the oil was tested at a local laboratory, they began treating Charlotte with small doses.

"We were pioneering the whole thing; we were guinea pigging Charlotte," according to Paige. *"This is a*

federally illegal substance. I was terrified to be honest with you."

Matt and Paige were very surprised at the results. Charlotte didn't have any seizures in the first hour, which was a positive first sign. And it just got better after that: the seizures were gone in about a week!

Charlotte's health has improved, and the seizures have become very infrequent, mostly happening only while she is sleeping. She has become physically active, being able to walk, ride a bicycle, and feed herself.

"I didn't hear her laugh for six months," Paige said. *"I didn't hear her voice at all, just her crying. I can't imagine that I would be watching her making these gains that she's making, doing the things that she's doing (without the medical marijuana). I don't take it for granted. Every day is a blessing."*

The strain of marijuana that Matt and Paige used for Charlotte is now called Charlotte's Web, and is being used by many other patients suffering from cancer, epilepsy, and other diseases.

Because of Charlotte's story, the spotlight has now been focused on CBD. Over the next few chapters, let's look at more characteristics of cannabidiol and why it is being regarded as a miracle compound.

Chapter Two: Health Benefits Of CBD

Key Takeaway: Ever since capturing headlines, CBD has been the toast of the town and become accepted in many sectors of society. Even among those who have traditionally rejected cannabis products because of the stigma of marijuana use as a recreational drug. In order to fully appreciate why medical researchers and scientists have continued to extol cannabidiol, one must take a look at the health benefits that have been derived or observed from CBD use.

The scientific and medical communities have made fascinating inroads into understanding the positive effects of cannabidiol in the human body. This has resulted into a growing acceptance of its various uses, and more research into how CBD in its many formulations and dosages can be prescribed to patients who are suffering from a wide range of ailments that have not been successfully or effectively relieved by other treatments.

Inflammation

Foremost of these benefits is the natural pain relief and anti-inflammation effects of CBD. While there are prescription and over-the-counter drugs used by many people to treat different kinds of pain, particularly chronic pain associated with illnesses, CBD offers a more natural way to alleviate pain. Currently, CBD is already being used to alleviate chronic pain in patients managing multiple sclerosis and fibromyalgia.

A 2012 study published in the Journal of Experimental Medicine found that CBD significantly inhibited inflammation and chronic pain in mice and rats. Researchers reported that "*systemic and intrathecal administration of cannabidiol (CBD), a major nonpsychoactive component of marijuana, and its modified derivatives significantly suppress chronic inflammatory and neuropathic pain without causing apparent analgesic tolerance in rodents."*

Nicotine

CBD is now being studied as potentially a solution for people who want to quit smoking cigarettes or are experiencing nicotine withdrawals.

Researchers from the Clinical Psychopharmacology Unit of the University College London published a pilot study in 2013 showing that smokers who used an inhaler containing CBD experienced reduced nicotine cravings and smoked about 40% fewer cigarettes. The control group with the placebo inhaler showed no significant difference in the number of cigarettes they smoked that week. Why is this result so remarkable? Because all subjects weren't even asked to stop or reduce their smoking!

Opioids

Another study found CBD to be a promising treatment for people who abuse opioids, due to its limited potential for abuse and ability to inhibit drug cravings.

For this study, the researchers investigated the effects of CBD on heroin addicts. On three consecutive days, they gave heroin-dependent individuals a dose of either CBD or a placebo. Next, they then showed them video cues that were either heroine related or neutral. At the same time, they measured any drug cravings that were induced by the cues. The result? In all subjects, CBD decreased their heroine cravings.

Epilepsy

CBD is increasingly being used to treat epilepsy, as we saw with the case of Charlotte Figi, discussed in the last chapter. A team of medical researchers and doctors published their findings in the June 2014 of Epilepsia which highlighted the anti-seizure properties of the compound, as well as its low risk of side effects. It appears that CBD has a positive effect on various neurological disorders linked to epilepsy, including neuronal injury, neurodegeneration, and psychiatric illnesses. However, they did note that more research and experiments need to be conducted for more conclusive findings.

In 2016, a team of research centers led by Orrin Devinsky of New York University Langone Medical Center published their findings based on a study of 162 patients with treatment-resistant epilepsy who were treated with a 99 percent CBD extract formula. The study, conducted over a 12-week period, was published in The Lancet Neurology and found reduced motor seizures in the patients. 2 percent of the subjects became completely seizure-free. Side effects included sleepiness, fatigue, and diarrhea, but only 3 percent of the patients had to discontinue due to the side effects.

Orrin Devinsky, a neurologist at New York University Langone Medical Center involved with this study, commented on the findings: *"I think, based on the evidence that we have, if a child has tried multiple standard drugs and the epilepsy is still severe and impairing quality of life, then the risks of trying CBD are low to modest at best."*

Cancer

Cancer is another disease for which CBD has been found to have positive effects. Notably, a review in the British Journal of Clinical Pharmacology from 2013 cited the cancer-blocking effects of cannabidiol, suppressing the growth and spread of cancer cells. Because it has low toxicity compared to other forms of cancer treatment available, researchers are calling for more studies into how CBD can be incorporated into medical treatment options available to cancer patients. And another study by the California Pacific Medical Center suggested that CBD kills the gene that causes breast cancer.

Anxiety Disorders

The potential benefits of CBD in treating a wide range of anxiety disorders has also recently come to light. Like all scientific research on the health effects of CBD, there are only a few studies. But the results of these studies are very promising.

For example, a review from Neurotherapeutics in 2015 by authors from New York University School of Medicine found that existing preclinical evidence strongly supports CBD as a treatment for generalized:

- anxiety disorder
- panic disorder
- social anxiety disorder
- obsessive–compulsive disorder, and
- post-traumatic stress disorder

when administered acutely.

It is believed that CBD can increase serotonin levels in the body, which tend to be low in people that suffer from anxiety.

Also, a 2011 study by a group of scientists who prescribed 600mg of CBD to people with Generalized Social Anxiety Disorder (SAD) found that participants had reduced levels of anxiety, cognitive impairment, and speech discomfort. *"These preliminary results indicate that a single dose of CBD can reduce the anxiety-enhancing effect provoked by SPST in SAD patients, indicating that this cannabinoid inhibits the fear of speaking in public, one of the main symptoms of the disorder,"* according to the study. *"Therefore, the effects of a single dose of CBD, observed in this study in the face of one of the main SAD's phobic stimuli, is a promising indication of a rapid onset of therapeutic effect in patients with SAD."*

Schizophrenia

CBD has also been shown to have antipsychotic effects, and may be useful for people suffering from schizophrenia. A study conducted by the University of Cologne in Germany enrolled 42 patients with exacerbated schizophrenia who were administered either cannabidiol or amisulpride, a common and highly potent antipsychotic drug.

Researchers remarked, *"Either treatment was safe and led to significant clinical improvement, but cannabidiol displayed a markedly superior side-effect profile. Moreover, cannabidiol treatment was accompanied by a significant increase in serum anandamide levels, which was significantly associated with clinical improvement. The results suggest that inhibition of anandamide deactivation may contribute to the antipsychotic effects of cannabidiol potentially representing a completely new mechanism in the treatment of schizophrenia."*

Also, another study showed that CBD had a superior effect than a placebo on 88 patients with schizophrenia who had failed to respond to any medication.

Type-1 Diabetes

Type-1 diabetes is another condition for which CBD may be helpful. In Type 1-diabetes, the cells in the pancreas are attacked by the body's immune system, causing inflammation. Research on non-obese diabetic mice, published by the Clinical Hemorheology and Microcirculation in 2016 and conducted by a team from Dalhousie University in Halifax, Nova Scotia, found that cannabidiol treatment significantly:

- reduced pancreatic inflammation, and
- lowered the incidence of diabetes

Acne

Because of its anti-inflammatory properties, studies are now also being conducted on the use of CBD in treating acne. A team of researchers from Europe and Japan published their study in the Journal of Clinical Investigation showing that CBD lowers the production of sebum in the body, thereby also reducing acne. The researchers concluded: *"Collectively, our findings suggest that, due to the combined lipostatic, antiproliferative, and antiinflammatory effects, CBD has potential as a promising therapeutic agent for the treatment of acne vulgaris."*

Alzheimer's Disease

Cannabidiol can also delay or prevent symptoms of Alzheimer's disease, according to initial research findings published in the Journal of Alzheimer's Disease. A research team from Australian universities studied Alzheimer's Disease transgenic mice treated with CBD for 8 months. Their findings?

They concluded that the study *"revealed a subtle impact of CBD on neuroinflammation, cholesterol, and dietary phytosterol retention, which deserves further investigation. This study is the first to demonstrate CBD's ability to prevent the development of a social recognition deficit in AD transgenic mice. Our findings provide the first evidence that CBD may have potential as a preventative treatment for AD with a particular relevance for symptoms of social withdrawal and facial recognition."*

Stimulates Appetite

If you have ever heard of cannabis users talking about getting the "munchies" when using the plant, it turns out there is actually a scientific reason behind it. CBD binds itself to the body's cannabinoid receptors and has been found to stimulate appetite, according to the National Cancer Institute. Cannabidiol is now being prescribed to patients who are going through chemotherapy or other forms of treatment that cause nausea and vomiting, limiting one's appetite. With controlled CBD use, a healthy appetite can be restored, ensuring that the body gets the nourishment it needs.

In a report made by a team from the Department of Psychology and Collaborative Neuroscience Program of the University of Guelph in Ontario, Canada, they cited recent studies showing the benefits of CBD dosage in patients who are experiencing various forms of nausea, vomiting, or eating disorders. According to the report *"evidence from animal experiments suggests that cannabinoids may be especially useful in treating the more difficult to control symptoms of nausea and anticipatory nausea in chemotherapy patients, which are less well controlled by the currently available conventional pharmaceutical agents. Although rats and mice are incapable of vomiting, they display a distinctive conditioned gaping response when re-exposed to cues (flavours or contexts) paired with a nauseating treatment."*

Other

Other conditions for which CBD has been used, prescribed, or suggested include:

- lupus
- osteoporosis
- Parkinson's disease, and
- several pediatric conditions.

While scientists and medical researchers caution that research into long-term positive effects of CBD are still inconclusive, the majority do believe that CBD has shown a lot of promise and merits the attention of the community in general.

Side Effects

Are there side effects when using CBD?

More studies need to be done in order to conclusively determine if there are harmful effects to the human body, especially after long-term use. However, initial experiments have shown that CBD is well-tolerated by the human body in dosages up to 1,500mg per day.

Some studies, particularly regarding Parkinson's Disease patients and CBD, have shown that cannabidiol may exacerbate tremors and muscle movements among patients, but the results are still early. On the other hand, many doctors are prescribing CBD to Parkinson's Disease sufferers because of its calming effect, so it seems any potential harmful effects are exceptions.

For now, the direction in which clinical trials and studies into the therapeutic effects of CBD is mostly positive, so it is definitely safe to consider as part of any treatment plan. Of course, it is always best to consult with your physician first and make sure that he or she is aware of any CBD products you are taking. CBD may interact with medication you are taking, so it is wise to let your doctor know and discuss options together.

If you live in a jurisdiction where medical or recreational cannabis has been legalized, you will likely find strains of the plant that have high concentrations of CBD versus THC, and as you will see in the next chapter, there are many different ways to consume CBD. The legalized cannabis industry in many parts of the world has opened up doors to consuming this miracle compound in different methods, so you can choose which method is most convenient for you and your needs.

Chapter Three: What Is CBD Hemp Oil?

Key Takeaway: There are a number of ways to consume CBD safely and legally, and the options will likely continue to grow as more studies are made on the benefits of CBD. CBD hemp oil is one of the simplest, most effective and readily available CBD formulations available to the average consumer today, regardless of geographic location.

Cannabis used to be a topic relegated to hushed conversations because of the general perception of it as an illicit substance prone to abuse.

However, growing acceptance of the plant, as well as overwhelming scientific evidence on the potential health and therapeutic benefits of the cannabis plant, have caused massive changes in legislation and mainstream acceptance of cannabis use across many parts of the world.

Disclaimer: Consult Your Physician Before Use

The decision on how to consume cannabidiol or CBD rests on:

- you and your physician's analysis of your health situation and how this compound can benefit you, as well as
- prevailing legal statutes in your locality regarding the sale, possession, and use of the cannabis plant and its derivative products.

Hemp Plant

It is important to note that while the cannabis plant has strains that are high in CBD, another option if you are looking for the therapeutic benefits of CBD would be to go for the hemp plant instead. Hemp-based CBD oil products are available in many parts of the world legally, and even available for orders and delivery in the United States. CBD hemp oil is extracted from high-CBD, low-THC hemp plants, and this oil is non-psychoactive.

The hemp plant itself contains trace amounts of THC, but unlike marijuana plants, the amount is much lower than the CBD contained, so there is no effect of being "high" or intoxicated. The CBD in hemp oil still contains the positive interactors that bind to the body's receptors, delivering the positive health benefits in a less controversial and socially acceptable package. In fact, in many areas of the world, CBD hemp oil products are sold in supermarkets and specialty stores, with no legal documents or medical cards necessary to purchase.

The hemp plant is imported into the United States for a variety of uses, including textile manufacturing, construction and building materials, paper products, and other nutritional supplements and food products, including the oil extraction. Both the hemp and marijuana plants come from the same cannabis plant species, but the difference is in their THC content. Whereas marijuana plants contain high levels of THC, hemp plants are made up of more CBD.

In the United States, it is illegal to grow hemp domestically because of existing laws that prohibit all varieties of the cannabis plant from being grown. Hemp is imported and must contain very low levels of THC. Efforts have been made in recent years, however, to reintroduce hemp domestically in light of continued scientific and medical explorations into its benefits, as well as the growing decriminalization and legalization of marijuana.

CBD Hemp Oil

So, what are your options for using CBD?

Perhaps the most potent would be the CBD hemp oil, bottled and sold in many stores.

CBD hemp oil in its purest, most potent form appears to be the most effective and with the quickest results. According to the 'Cannabidiol Daily' blog, if you want to get the most from CBD, CBD hemp oil is the way to go:

"CBD concentrated oils contain the strongest dose of CBD compared to other CBD products, with different oils ranging from 50-200mg of CBD per serving. CBD oils can be administered orally by swallowing the oil or allowing it to be absorbed through the inner linings of the mouth and tongue (sublingual)."

You do want to make sure that the CBD hemp oil you are purchasing contains no other additives, and has been rigorously tested for quality. Pure CBD hemp oil can be ingested.

Tinctures

Another way to consume CBD is through tinctures, sprays, inhalers, or liquid drops. These oil products would be better alternatives if you do not need to consume CBD in large amounts of its purest form, unlike the bottled varieties, or for younger patients. Tinctures, sprays, and liquid drops are easier to control and you can more efficiently manage dosage as well. If you are going about your day and want your CBD fix, a tincture or spray would be a great option.

Topical

There are also CBD-based topical products widely available. CBD-based topical creams, salves, ointments, and lotions have been used for soothing muscle pain, reducing inflammation and soreness, and even alleviating pain from arthritis, nerve damage, back pain, tendonitis, gout, dry skin, and other external conditions.

Vaporizing

Another way to consume CBD is through vaporizing. You can purchase vaporizer pens from smoke shops and other stores in your community, and vaporize CBD oils without the adverse effects of smoking. Vaporizer pens are especially useful if you are always travelling. You can just bring the CBD oil and the vaporizer with you, and you can get your CBD fix any time you want.

Capsules / Pills

CBD capsules and pills are also becoming quite popular. In many herbal stores and food supplement retail centers, CBD hemp oil capsules and pills are sold alongside other more popular nutritional supplements, organic products, and herbal treatments. Generally speaking, CBD-based capsules and pills are not as potent as the liquid form, so make sure you are getting a product with the least additives and processing to ensure you are still getting the amount of CBD you need.

As you can see, there are different ways to reap the various health benefits of CBD. For many, CBD Hemp Oil is their best option. But the important thing to consider is to find a method that works best for your lifestyle, your needs, and your day-to-day schedule. You may even find that a combination of two or more CBD consumption methods, depending on the time of day and the activity you are involved in, would be best for your personal situation.

Chapter Four: Factors for Purchasing CBD Hemp Oil

Key Takeaway: *When buying CBD Hemp Oil, make sure you take into account factors like cannabidiol strength, purity, whether the hemp is produced organically, information transparency, and the price.*

What factors should you look at when purchasing CBD hemp oil products? There are a few aspects you should always consider.

Cannabidiol Strength

The first things to take into account is the cannabidiol strength. CBD strength refers to the amount or percentage of CBD compared to the hemp oil. Also related to this is the volume of CBD in the product.

This can be found in the product labels, usually shown as percentages of the total product volume.

CBD strength is important to take note of because you would not want to start off with very large doses of CBD right away, especially if you are new to this compound. The average dosage for an adult would be between 1 mg to 2 mg per day during the first week. Monitor how your body reacts to the CBD hemp oil product first, and then gradually increase as needed.

Purity

The second factor to look at when purchasing CBD hemp oil products is their purity. As already mentioned, some CBD hemp oil products may contain additives, preservatives, or solvents. Not all of these additives or preservatives are harmful, of course. But you do want to make the clear distinction and know what is in the CBD hemp oil product, especially if you plan on ingesting the product.

In February 2016, the U.S. Food and Drug Administration issued a warning after having found that several CBD products on the market did not have the appropriate amount of CBD levels in their items, contrary to their claims. "*It is important to note that these products are not approved by FDA for the diagnosis, cure, mitigation, treatment, or prevention of any disease. Consumers should beware purchasing and using any such products,*" according to the FDA warning.

Companies and products that were cited in the FDA warning included:

- Cali Stores (CBDy CBD Supplement Tincture, Hermosa Farm CannaHoney w/ CBD)
- Dose of Nature (Nano CBD Shooter, Red Strap Hemp Extract 250 – Coconut Oil)
- Green Garden Gold (CBD - Regular CBD-Oil, CBD - Strawberry Jam CBD-Oil)
- Healthy Hemp Oil (Herbal Renewals CBD Hemp Oil Supplement, Herbal Renewals 25% CBD

Hemp Oil Gold Label, PLUS+CBD Oil Balm, Hempotion Cannabidiol CBD Concentrate, Entourage Occam's Razor)

- Michigan Herbal Remedies (Bluebird Botanicals Bulletproof CBD Blend, US Hemp Wholesale 25% CBD Hemp Oil Supplement Gold Label, Endoca Hemp Oil, Alternate Vape LUV-A-BULL, Tasty Hemp Oil - Tasty Drops Hemp Oil Supplement, Tasty Vape Hemp Oil - Just Peachy, PLUS+CBD Oil Spray)
- PainBomb (iHempCBD Filtered CBD Hemp Oil, PainBomb + CBD), and Sana Te Premium Oils (CBD Oil - 25.2% CBD)

And there are more on the list.

What does this mean for you? If you are purchasing CBD hemp oils and products, make sure that it is coming from a legitimate, legally recognized, and trusted source. Check out reviews or feedback from previous users, and find out as much as you can about the manufacturer you are purchasing from.

Choose Organic

If possible, you would also want to look for CBD hemp oil products made from organic hemp products, or hemp products sourced from plants that have not been laced with herbicides, pesticides, and other chemical fertilizers. A good indicator to look for is whether the CBD hemp oil product is derived from certified organic industrial hemp.

Information Transparency

Information transparency is also a must when you are selecting which CBD hemp oil products to patronize. Oversight for CBD hemp oil products is still largely being underwritten, so you can protect yourself as a consumer by making sure you are only purchasing from companies that are transparent about their products' laboratory test results, formulations, and certifications. This way, you have all the information you need on whether the CBD content advertised is correct, the THC content is low, etc.

Price

Price is a factor in many of our purchasing decisions, and in buying your CBD hemp oil products you would also want to get the best products at the best possible prices. That said, you should be aware that due to the refinement processes and procurement methods that take place in order to produce the best CBD hemp oil extracts, those with purer, higher quality CBD content will likely be more expensive than their counterparts. Do not hesitate to pay more for better quality.

Chapter Five: The Various Kinds Of Hemp Oil

Key Takeaway: Not all hemp oils are the same. If you are looking specifically to benefit from the health effects of CBD, you should be aware of the other types of hemp oils and how different they are from what we know as CBD hemp oil. This avoids confusion, misunderstanding, and negative experiences.

Aside from the different CBD hemp oil products available in the market today, you should also be aware of the *varieties* of hemp oil that are available today. Especially if you are looking to purchase CBD hemp oil as is.

It can be quite confusing for the uninitiated or those who are newly researching CBD hemp oil when they see other types of hemp oils, only to find that the intended effects and/or uses are not the same.

Hemp Seed Oil

For instance, if you come across hemp seed oil, whether pure, processed, or in derivatives, you may easily confuse this with CBD hemp oil which we have extensively discussed so far. While both CBD hemp oil and hemp seed oil come from the same hemp plant, they are fundamentally different.

As its name suggests, hemp seed oil is extracted from the seeds of the hemp plant. You will easily distinguish unrefined, cold-pressed hemp seed oil because of its green color and nutty flavor. On the other hand, refined hemp seed oil has a clear, transparent color, and with very little flavor. In fact, refined hemp seed oil is more used for body care products, lubricants, plastic manufacturing, and fuel products.

Hemp Essential Oil

Another hemp oil you may see in the market is the hemp essential oil, which you also should not confuse for CBD hemp oil. Hemp essential oil is extracted from the upper flowers and leaves of the plant itself using steam distillation. Hemp essential oil is distinguishable by its pale yellow to light green coloring and a strong therapeutic aroma.

Hemp essential oil is quite expensive because of the amount of hemp foliage needed to make just an ounce of the oil. Also, it does not contain any amounts of THC or CBD. You will find hemp essential oils mixed into massage oils, scented candles, aromatherapy products, and other items for relaxation, health, and wellness.

Want To Buy CBD Hemp Oil? Make Sure You Inform Yourself!

While these different types of hemp oil products do have their own purposes and effective uses, they are characteristically different from CBD hemp oil itself, and if you are looking to glean the health benefits of CBD particularly from the hemp plant, you will not find these benefits in any of the other hemp products other than CBD hemp oil itself. In fact, CBD is not even present in hemp essential oils, and if present in hemp seed oil can be in very small trace amounts only.

This distinction is important to discuss. As more and more consumers become aware of the positive uses and effects of CBD hemp oil, they may turn to the Web or their local retail stores for information on where to get CBD hemp oils and products. However, they may come across wrong, misleading, or confusing information that results in a negative experience overall.

CBD hemp oil is an altogether different product from the essential oils and hemp seed oils that are also marketed commercially, so be aware of the distinctions.

If you want to be absolutely sure that you are getting the correct and the best CBD hemp oil products, perhaps a good way to start looking locally would be herbal or organic stores or medical marijuana dispensaries in your area. Typically, store owners and employees in these establishments would already know the basic differences, and would be able to point you in the right direction or refer you to the best products available.

Chapter Six: How To Make CBD Hemp Oil

Key Takeaway: While CBD hemp oil is available to consumers, you also have the option of extracting the oil yourself from the hemp plant. Know what methods to use, and which ones are most suitable or realistic for your lifestyle.

Do-it-yourself projects offer you more hands-on involvement and the freedom to control as much of the intended results and the overall process as you are willing to. Of course, the responsibilities and tasks would also be magnified if you take on a project yourself rather than relying on readily-available sources or methods, but it does come with the satisfaction of knowing that you have more control over the outcome.

Perhaps you are interested in making your own CBD hemp oil and would like to know:

- how this is done
- what the required equipment and processes would be, and
- where to source the necessary supplies.

The great thing about deciding to extract your own CBD hemp oil these days is that there is a growing CBD enthusiast community already online and in localities all around the world. This means you can readily get information from people who are already involved in the process and can give you the needed information and resources.

High-Grade Food-Safe Alcohol

One way to extract CBD hemp oil is with the use of high-grade food-safe alcohol. This process works best if your plan is to extract edible CBD hemp oil for direct use, drops, or for mixing with food. Here is a simple process for extracting CBD hemp oil:

You will need:

- Around 30g of ground buds or 60-100g of ground, dried trim or shake
- 4 liters of grain alcohol or other food-safe, high-grade alcohol
- Equipment
- Glass or ceramic mixing bowl
- Fine strainer i.e. cheesecloth, sieve, or nylon stockings
- Catchment container
- Double boiler (you can utilize two fitted saucepans or pots stacked together with enough space between them)
- Wooden spoon, silicon spatula, funnel, plastic syringe

Arrange your equipment carefully and ensure that your working area is clean, sterilized, and ready for the procedure. Completely cover the plant material in the mixing bowl with alcohol and stir for 3-5 minutes with the wooden spoon to bring out the resin. Check to make sure that the bowl can easily contain both the raw material and the solvent.

Next, filter the liquid into the sieve and collect this first raw extraction into the catchment container, squeezing out as much of the fluid as you can. The stirring and filtering process can be repeated with another batch of the solvent to extract as much compounds as possible from the plant matter.

After this, pour the strained liquid into the double boiler and heat until bubbles start to appear. Let all the alcohol evaporate without changing the temperature.

Keep the heat at minimum or turn it on and off occasionally, because the mixture has to keep gently bubbling for about 15-30 minutes. Keep stirring and don't let the liquid get excessively hot. As the alcohol evaporates, mix the solution and scrape the bowl with the silicon spatula.

Now, carefully transfer the concentrated oil into a storage bottle or dosage containers before it cools off and thickens. You can draw the CBD oil into plastic syringes or pour it into small airtight containers for storage. Dosage amounts can be portioned off by squeezing small amounts of oil out from the syringe, or by using toothpicks and small spoons. The CBD oil extraction with the grain alcohol method is one of the safest and simplest processes, and its products are great for direct consumption.

Mix Hemp Extract With Virgin Coconut Oil or Sweet Almond Oil

If you are looking to make your CBD hemp oil an herbal ointment instead, you can try this process which mixes the hemp extract with virgin coconut oil or sweet almond oil:

You will need:

- 1 Cup of a high-quality virgin coconut oil or sweet almond oil
- 14 grams of organic hemp CBD buds and leaves

With the use of a coffee grinder, grind the buds, stems, and leaves of the hemp plant.

Place the hemp in a small glass canning jar and cover it with the oil, then tightly replace the lid. Put a washrag in a small saucepan and place the jar in the saucepan. Pour about two or three inches of water in the pan. Heat the water to just below boiling point. Heat the water for about 3 hours. If the water level in the pot decreases due to evaporation, add some water to make sure the pot does not dry out. Shake the jar a few times every hour.

After 3 hours, turn off the stove and cover the pot with a towel. Let the jar cool for another 3 hours, then repeat the process. Now let the jar sit in the pot, covered with the towel overnight. Repeat the process for the 3 days, if possible. The oil should actually be ready to use after one day but the longer you repeat this process, the stronger your oil extract will be. Finally, strain the oil and herbs through a cheesecloth into another glass jar for storage. Ensure that the cloth is squeezed so you can get each drop of the hemp oil extract. Remember that this is not for ingestion, but more for topical use.

Sourcing

Sourcing your hemp is another consideration for these do-it-yourself CBD hemp oil extraction efforts. If you live in the United States, growing hemp is still largely illegal due to laws that prohibit the growing of cannabis plants, although changes are coming rapidly and these regulations are already under review. In the meantime, hemp in the United States is imported and must have low levels of THC.

Otherwise, if you live in a jurisdiction where you can legally grow your own hemp plants, then you already have the sourcing part of the process taken care of. Hemp is actually one of the fastest growing plants out there, so if you are able to grow your own hemp plants in your backyard, you will not have to wait a very long time to be able to see the yield. Industrial hemp has a growth cycle of 12-14 weeks.

If you reside in the northern hemisphere, the best months to plant hemp would be between March and May. For those in the southern hemisphere, it is best to plant your hemp seeds between September and November. There are about 26 varieties of hemp with low levels of THC certified by the European Union. These varieties or cultivars have less than 0.2% THC content, and between 1% to 5% cannabidiol content. Importing of hemp in the United States requires the THC content to be below 0.3%.

For the best hemp yields, you should have soil that is deep and rich in humus, and dense with nutrients.

Hemp can withstand cold temperatures, but requires a lot of heat and water to full maturation. It is also worth noting that hemp has a positive effect on the soil in which it is grown, which means you can use the soil for planting a different crop and alternate with hemp growing.

Before making any major decisions on whether to proceed with your own CBD hemp oil extraction efforts, as well as whether or not to grow your own hemp plants, you should first be aware of the legal status of this plant in the area where you live. In the next chapter, we will take a look at the legal ramifications for you to study.

Chapter Seven: Legal Aspects Concerning CBD Hemp Oil

__Key Takeaway__: The legal language surrounding CBD hemp oil products continues to change with each passing day. What basic knowledge should you possess, especially if you live in the United States?

Perhaps you are concerned about the legal aspect of CBD hemp oil products. You will be pleased to know that in the United States, it is legal to use CBD oil products as long as they are derived from the hemp plant's stalks or seeds, not the flowers. Also, THC restrictions must be met.

Current Status: Legal to Sell and Buy CBD Hemp Oil

First, let's look at the good news: CBD hemp oil and the various products and derivatives based on or containing CBD hemp oil can be imported and sold in the United States, as long as they contain less than 0.3% THC.

Importers and manufacturers are legally importing CBD hemp oil products by complying with the U.S. Controlled Substances Act of 1970, which allows non-THC producing cannabis plants and products to be imported.

In order to comply with this Act, importers and manufacturers do not produce their own CBD oil. Instead, their CBD oil is produced in European countries, where it is legal to grow hemp. Then they import the CBD hemp oil to the U.S., where it is packaged and sold.

This workaround has enabled these companies to sell their CBD hemp oil products and compete with other forms of CBD extracts that are only available for sale in medical marijuana states.

You can CBD Hemp Oil online, or walk into herbal or organic stores, even many supermarkets and grocery stores, and find CBD hemp oils, extracts, vapors, ointments, salves, capsules, gum, and other products.

You will find many sellers and producers based all over the world who manufacture a wide range of these CBD hemp oil products. In the United States, they are strictly controlled and tested for quality, as well as to ensure that they pass legal requirements, but you do not need any special documentation or medical marijuana card in order to purchase CBD hemp oil. They can even be delivered straight to your residence.

What About Growing Your Own Hemp?

As far as growing your own hemp, you may find this more promising but not completely without barriers at this time, if you live in the United States. In 2014, the Federal Farm Bill was passed which allows farmers residing in states with industrial hemp legislation to grow and harvest hemp, as long as this is done in conjunction with their state agriculture departments, primarily for research pilot programs only.

While it is initially only for research purposes, farmers are pressing on amidst the challenges, such as Will and Ally Cabaniss. They moved from Florida to Colorado to start a 20-acre hemp farm after the 2014 Farm Bill was passed. "*Every day brings something new and different,*" Will explained in a 2016 article published in the Pittsburgh Tribune-Review. "*Right now we're just building data for the industry, seeing what works and what doesn't.*"

Farmers looking to be part of the pilot research and development programs for hemp farming have to reside in one of the 29 states that have authorized hemp research, and also contend with the still expensive prices of imported hemp seeds, currently running at around $5 to $10 per seed.

Why Are There Legal Restrictions On CBD?

Hemp (which, if you remember, contains a lot of CBD) has been used for thousands of years. As a matter of fact, it is considered one of the oldest domesticated crops we know of. Hemp has been used for textiles and paper, and its seeds and flowers for health foods and organic body care. Henry Ford even considered hemp ethanol as fuel for one of his first cars. If you go to YouTube, you can even find old footage of Henry Ford's Hemp Plastic Car!

So, that begs the questions: why did the U.S. government decide to ban cultivation of hemp?

Because the crop is so versatile that it poses a threat to powerful industries such as cotton, plastic, paper, and petroleum. They had – and have! – a financial interest in the prohibition of hemp, and have lobbied strongly for it since the 1930s. This resulted in the Marijuana Tax Act of 1937, and later the Controlled Substances Act of 1970. This legislation makes it illegal to grow any cannabis plant, including hemp, in the United States.

The lobby on the psychoactive effects of marijuana has been so successful that most people don't even know anymore that hemp is not the same as marijuana, and is actually a very versatile crop that can be used for many different things that would enrich our lives, improve our health, and possibly even make the world a better place.

Good News: Industrial Hemp Farming Act

The biggest and most promising step so far in the United States toward legalizing hemp is the bill for the

Industrial Hemp Farming Act, which was introduced in 2015. This bill, sponsored by a group of lawmakers from both the Republican and Democratic parties, would end all federal bans on hemp production in the United States.

"The federal ban on hemp has been a waste of taxpayer dollars that ignores science, suppresses innovation, and subverts the will of states that have chosen to incorporate this versatile crop into their economies," according to Rep. Jared Polis (D-Colo.), one of the bill's co-sponsors, in the press release for the bill. *"I am hopeful that Congress will build on last year's progress on hemp research and pilot programs by passing the Industrial Hemp Farming Act to allow this historical American crop to once again thrive on our farmlands."*

The bill seeks to correct current measures that make the U.S. the largest industrialized country that prohibits domestic hemp production, all while being the largest consumer of hemp products in the world today.

Bad News: DEA Ruling – CBD is a Schedule 1 Drug

Where the Industrial Hemp Farming Act is good news, there is also some bad news coming from the Drug Enforcement Administration (DEA). In January 2017, in a ruling that specifically targeted CBD oil products, the DEA ruled that CBD is a Schedule 1 drugs: "*Meaning an extract containing one or more cannabinoids that has been derived from any plant of the genus Cannabis, other than the separated resin (whether crude or purified) obtained from the plant.*"

This ruling has been heavily criticized, for example by Robert Hoban, a Colorado cannabis attorney and adjunct professor of law at the University of Denver. When interviewed for an article published on Leafly, he pointed out that the ruling may not even be lawful: "*The DEA can only carry out the law, they cannot create it. Here they're purporting to create an entirely new category called 'marijuana extracts,' and by doing so wrest control over all cannabinoids. They want to call all cannabinoids illegal. But they don't have the authority to do that."*

It is very likely that this ruling will eventually be challenged in court, should the DEA actively enforce it.

What Will The Future Bring?

Until it is passed, pro-hemp activists and information disseminators are continuing to trumpet the benefits of hemp in its many forms, including CBD hemp oil and the therapeutic effects.

It seems like an uphill battle still for those in the United States who may want to grow their own industrial hemp, whether it is for their personal consumption or for commercial purposes. If you reside in other countries, however, such as:

- The Netherlands
- France
- Romania
- Lithuania
- Ukraine
- Switzerland
- Russia
- Canada
- Australia
- New Zealand
- Japan
- Korea
- Turkey
- Thailand, or
- Chile,

among others, you can look into growing your own hemp plants for your extraction purposes, and perhaps even start a thriving business especially as demand for this compound increases worldwide.

For those in the United States, do not let the barriers on domestic hemp production or farming hinder you from benefiting from the many wonderful health and wellness effects of CBD hemp oil. It is still legal to import hemp in the United States, and CBD hemp oils and products in many forms are legal to purchase.

Conclusion

Thanks again for taking the time to read this book!

You should now have a good understanding of cannabidiol and CBD hemp oil products, and be able to make reasonable decisions regarding its use and whether it is a viable option for you to consider in your own journey towards better health and wellness.

As you have read, the discussions surrounding CBD products continue to evolve over the years, and all signs point to these discussions continuing unabated as the scientific and medical communities continue to perform more tests and unravel more of the wonders of this exceptional compound known as cannabidiol.

What is important at this stage is to keep an open mind and be willing to learn from different sources of information. As what is known about CBD and its products continue to grow over time, you can expect more innovations and changes in this segment of the market.

In many ways, the increased acceptance of hemp for consumer use, particularly as it pertains to domestic production in the United States, has been greatly impacted by the openness of many who have tried it and came forward with the positive effects of CBD in their lives, especially in relation to the treatment and alleviation of many serious and chronic illnesses in which modern medicine has been lacking.

But it also cannot be denied that the shift in perception in favor of CBD has also been greatly influenced by the growing movement among much of the world today to find more natural, sustainable ways to treat diseases and reduce the toxic effects of drugs. While there are many prescription medications and therapies that have been formulated to help in managing diabetes, cancer, Alzheimer's, Parkinson's, epilepsy, and mental disorders, they often also have adverse or toxic side effects.

CBD, as it has been shown in many research trials, is absorbed well by the human body and has very little side effects. This makes cannabidiol one of the more exciting components of medical research to watch out for in the coming years as more trials are conducted into this natural compound.

BONUS CHAPTER: A Brief History of Cannabis

*This is a bonus chapter from my book '**DIY CANNABIS EXTRACTS 101**: The Essential And Easy Beginner's Cannabis Cookbook On How To Make Medical Marijuana Extracts At Home.'*

Enjoy!

***

Key Takeaway*: The use of the cannabis plant (hemp) for woven fabric dates back over 11,000 years ago. Its first recorded use of ingestion is in 2737 BC, when the Chinese Emperor advocated is as medication. Cannabis extracts have a shorter history, it only started in the late 20th century. However, it* *has seen a quick rise in popularity, especially among those interested in its medicinal qualities.*

The history of the cannabis plant is a long and interesting one that dates back well into pre-historical times. The hemp plants durability and ability to grow literally anywhere under any conditions is what has made it such a resilient product throughout history.

Cannabis: A Journey Through The Ages

It is believed that the first woven forms of fabric were in fact used from the hemp plant, over 11,000 years ago. But in terms of its actual ingestion, the first recorded use can be traced back to 2737 B.C.E. This first use was by the Chinese Emperor Shen Nung who advocated it as a medication for gout, malaria and rheumatism, among other things. Although it was also used for intoxication purposes, it was its medical proficiencies that were considered most important.

And indeed, marijuana has been used consistently by a range of different cultures across the globe for thousands of years, from the Egyptians who used it to treat glaucoma and inflammations, right on through to the Persians who listed it as one of the most important medical plants.

It didn't find its way into the white America's until its introduction to Jamestown in 1611. And even then it was regaled for its medical uses above its hallucinogenic properties. Cannabis enjoyed immense, and legal, popularity in America for several hundred years in fact. It wasn't until the 1930s that a taboo grew around it and even still, it wasn't until The Controlled Substance Act of 1970 that it became classed as a schedule 1 drug and became completely illegal across the board.

It might be argued that there has been a resurgence in the popularity of marijuana of late, especially where it pertains to its medical functions. Because at the end of the day, once you eliminate the recreational properties that marijuana is most popular for, it's also an amazing healer and can be used for a range of different medical purposes.

Cannabis As A Medical Treatment

As mentioned above, cannabis has been in use as a form of medicine since at least 2737 BC. In the U.S. especially, its medical properties are starting to be preached more and more regularly as more states move towards legalising marijuana for both medical and recreational use.

It is generally believed that the cannabis plant has two active chemicals that can be harnessed for medical value. These are cannabidiol (CBD) and tetrahydrocannabinol (THC). CBD is believed to be able to impact the brain without inducing a high state where THC is believed to have the ability to reduce pain and inflammations. Together, and where properly applied, they can work wonders.

Examples of ailments that marijuana has been known to either cure or have a significant impact on include glaucoma, epilepsy, anxiety, Alzheimer's disease, multiple sclerosis and even some forms of cancer.

The reason that there are so many presumptions around medicinal marijuana, rather than cold hard facts, is due to its classification as a schedule 1 drug. Under law, drugs that fall into this category can't even be studied in order to confirm their medical benefits; at least not at the federal level.

But even so, most agree that its applications are endless and what's more, with the recent insurgence of cannabis extracts, these treatments are becoming readily available to more and more people.

A Brief History Of Extraction

Unlike cannabis itself, cannabis extracts have a very brief history. There are of course stories that have emerged from Word War II scientific experiments that utilized THC extraction for mind-bending experiments. And in 1937, the book 'Cannabis Alchemy: The Art of Modern Hashmaking,' was published. It gives a brief overview of how to make hash 'honey oil.' But it wasn't until well into the 1990s that extracting really took off.

The extracting boom is generally credited to the online psychoactive library Erowid which, in 1999, put out an article titled 'Hash Honey Oil Technique.' This was the first detailed description of using butane oil to extract hash oil. Although it was very dangerous and a little on the amateur side, it did give birth to what is now known as the 'closed loop system' of extraction.

I'm getting ahead of myself here, but as a preview of what is to come: a closed loop extraction is one in which butane is run over the marijuana plant, solvating the THC chemical from it. It then enters a collection chamber and evaporates the butane chemical, leaving you with a pure THC product, or 'extract.' This form of extraction is used across the board when it comes to butane extraction and is responsible for the rise in popularity of cannabis extracts.

So, what is a cannabis extract exactly? We'll look at that next!

***

This is the end of this bonus chapter.

Want to continue reading?

Then go to Amazon and search for 'DIY Cannabis Extracts 101'.

Hope to see you there!

Did You Like This Book?

If you enjoyed this book, I would like to ask you for a favor. Would you be kind enough to share your thoughts and post a review of this book on Amazon?

Just a few sentences would already be really helpful!

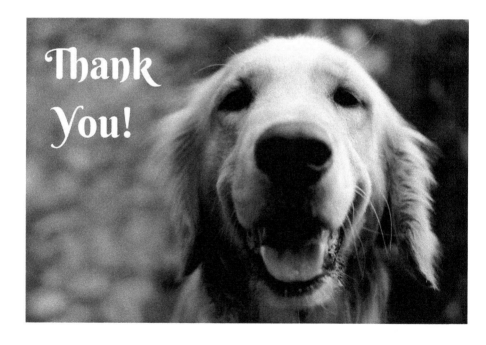

Your voice is important for this book to reach as many people as possible.

The more reviews this book gets, the more parents will be able to find it and learn about the wonderful health effects of CBD Hemp Oil.

Thank you again for reading this book and good luck with applying everything you have learned!

I'm rooting for you...

By The Same Author

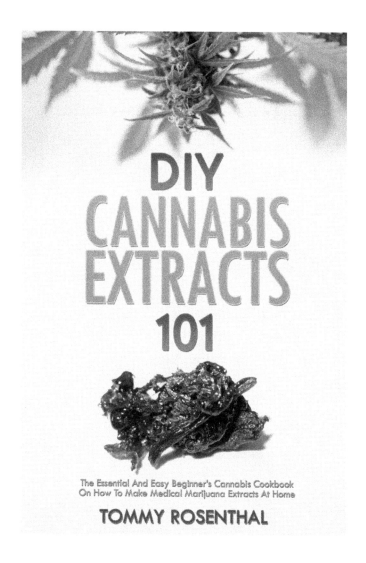

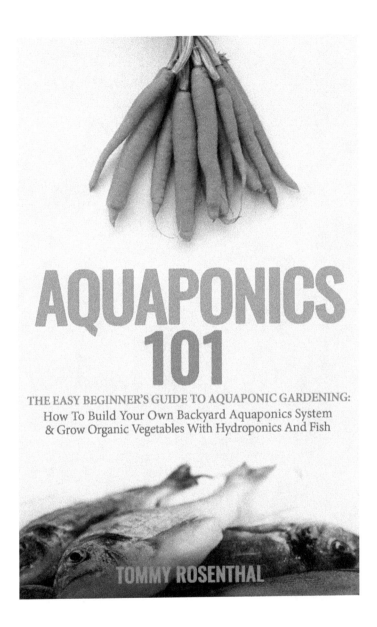

AQUAPONICS
101

THE EASY BEGINNER'S GUIDE TO AQUAPONIC GARDENING:
How To Build Your Own Backyard Aquaponics System
& Grow Organic Vegetables With Hydroponics And Fish

TOMMY ROSENTHAL

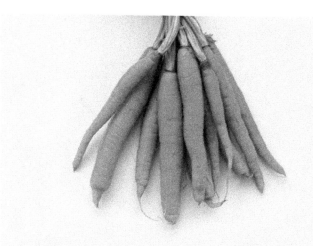

HYDROPONICS
101

THE EASY BEGINNER'S GUIDE TO HYDROPONIC GARDENING:
Learn How To Build a Backyard Hydroponics System
for Homegrown Organic Fruit, Herbs and Vegetables

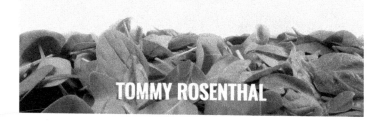

TOMMY ROSENTHAL

9 781986 144223